CROCK POT RECIPES 2021

EASY CROCK POT RECIPES FOR BEGINNERS

CECILIA HAMPTON

Table of Contents

Hearty Sausage Sandwiches

(Ready in about 6 hours | Servings 6)

Ingredients

- 8 links fresh sausages

- 1 cup beef broth

- 4 cups spaghetti sauce

- 1 chili pepper, minced

- 1 red bell pepper, sliced

- 1 green bell pepper, sliced

- 1 cup spring onions, chopped

- 1 heaping tablespoon fresh parsley

- 1 heaping tablespoon fresh cilantro

- 6 cocktail buns, split lengthwise

Directions

1. In a crock pot, place the sausage links, beef broth, spaghetti sauce, chili pepper, bell peppers and spring onions. Add parsley and cilantro. Stir to combine.

2. Cover with a lid; cook on Low for 6 hours. Serve on cocktail rolls and enjoy!

Country Smoked Sausages

(Ready in about 6 hours | Servings 6)

Ingredients

- 1 tablespoon extra-virgin olive oil

- 6 green onions, sliced

- 1 yellow bell pepper, sliced

- 1 red bell pepper, sliced

- 4 garlic cloves, smashed

- 2 pounds smoked sausage

- 1 (28-ounce) can tomatoes, diced

- 1 teaspoon salt

- 1/2 teaspoon ground black pepper

- 1/2 teaspoon red pepper flakes, crushed

- Mustard for garnish

Directions

1. In a large skillet, heat olive oil over medium flame. Sauté onions, bell peppers, garlic and sausages until vegetables are tender and sausages are lightly browned. Transfer to the crock pot.

2. Add tomatoes, salt, black pepper and red pepper.

3. Cook on low approximately 6 hours. Serve with your favourite mustard.

Must-Eat Beef Tacos

(Ready in about 8 hours | Servings 6)

Ingredients

- 1 ½ pounds beef chuck roast, boneless

- 1 large-sized red onion, sliced

- 1 cup beef stock

- 1 (16-ounce) jar taco sauce

- 12 taco shells

- 2 cucumbers, thinly sliced

- 2 ripe tomatoes, sliced

Directions

1. Lay beef chuck roast and sliced onion in a crock pot. Pour in beef stock and taco sauce.

2. Cook on LOW for 8 hours or overnight.

3. In the morning, cut beef into shreds.

4. Fill taco shells with shredded beef; add cucumber and tomato and serve!

Oatmeal with Prunes and Apricots

(Ready in about 8 hours | Servings 4)

Ingredients

- 1 cup steel cut oats

- 4 ½ cups water

- 1/2 teaspoon grated ginger

- 1/2 teaspoon allspice

- 1/2 teaspoon ground cinnamon

- 1⁄2 teaspoon salt

- 3 tablespoons butter

- 1⁄2 cup prunes

- 1/2 cup dried apricots

- Maple syrup, to taste

Directions

1. Put all ingredients into a crock pot.

2. Cover and cook on low-heat setting approximately 8 hours.

3. Serve with milk and some extra fruit if desired.

Muesli with Coconut and Peanuts

(Ready in about 2 hours | Servings 12)

Ingredients

- 4 cups rolled oats

- 4 cups water

- 1 teaspoon allspice

- 1/4 teaspoon turmeric

- 1 cup wheat germ

- 1 cup baking natural bran

- 1⁄2 cup shredded coconut, unsweetened

- 1⁄2 cup brown sugar

- 4 tablespoons butter, melted

- 1 teaspoon almond extract

- 2 tablespoons pumpkin seeds

- Peanuts for garnish

Directions

1. Add all of the ingredients, except peanuts, to your crock pot.

2. Cover with a lid; cook on high-heat setting approximately 2 hours, stirring twice. Divide among 12 serving bowls, scatter chopped peanuts on top and serve!

Cheese Steak Sandwiches

(Ready in about 8 hours | Servings 8)

Ingredients

- 1 pound round steak, thinly sliced

- 1 cup onions, sliced

- 1 green bell pepper, sliced

- 1 cup beef stock

- 1 clove garlic, minced

- 2 tablespoon red dry wine

- 1 tablespoon Worcestershire sauce

- 1 teaspoon celery seeds

- 1/2 teaspoon salt

- 1/4 teaspoon ground black pepper

- 8 hamburger buns

- 1 cup mozzarella cheese, shredded

Directions

1. Combine all of the ingredients, except buns and cheese, in your crock pot.

2. Cover and cook on low 6 to 8 hours.

3. Make sandwiches with buns, prepared meat mixture and cheese. Serve warm and enjoy!

Beer Brats with Mushrooms and Onion

(Ready in about 8 hours | Servings 8)

Ingredients

- 8 fresh bratwurst

- 2 (12-ounce) 3 bottles beer

- 1 cup mushrooms, sliced

- 2-3 cloves garlic, minced

- 1 red onion, sliced

- 1 red bell pepper, sliced

- 1 teaspoon sea salt

- 1/4 teaspoon ground black pepper

- 1 teaspoon minced poblano pepper

- 8 hot dog buns

Directions

1. Combine all ingredients, except buns, in a crock pot.

2. Cook, covered, on low 6 to 8 hours.

3. Serve cooked bratwurst and veggies in buns. Add mustard, catsup and sour cream if desired.

Yummy Sausage and Sauerkraut Sandwiches

(Ready in about 8 hours | Servings 6)

Ingredients

- 6 fresh sausages of choice

- 1 medium-sized onion, chopped

- 1 cup sauerkraut

- 1 small-sized apple, peeled, cored and thinly sliced

- 1 teaspoon caraway seeds

- 1/2 cup chicken broth

- Salt to taste

- 1/2 teaspoon ground black pepper

- 6 hot dog buns

- Catsup for garnish

- Mustard for garnish

Directions

1. Lay sausages in a crock pot. Then place onion, sauerkraut, apple, caraway seeds, chicken broth, salt and black pepper.

2. Cook, covered, on low 6 to 8 hours.

3. Make sandwiches with buns and serve with catsup and mustard.

Christmas Sausage Casserole

(Ready in about 8 hours | Servings 8)

Ingredients

- Non-stick cooking spray butter flavour

- 1 (26-ounce) package frozen hash brown potatoes, thawed

- 1 zucchini, thinly sliced

- 1 cup whole milk

- 10 eggs, beaten

- 1 teaspoon sea salt

- 1/4 teaspoon crushed red pepper flakes

- 1/4 teaspoon ground black pepper

- 1 teaspoon caraway seeds

- 1 tablespoon ground mustard

- 2 cups sausages

- 2 cups Cheddar cheese, shredded

Directions

1. Grease a crock pot with non-stick cooking spray. Spread hash browns to cover the bottom of the crock pot. Then lay zucchini slices.

2. In a medium-sized bowl, whisk milk, eggs, salt, red pepper, black pepper, caraway seeds, and ground mustard.

3. Heat a cast-iron skillet over medium flame. Next, cook the sausages until they are browned and crumbly, about 6 minutes; discard grease.

4. Lay sausage on zucchini layer, then spread Cheddar cheese. Pour egg-milk mixture over cheese layer.

5. Cook on low for 6 to 8 hours. Serve warm with some extra mustard.

Overnight Sausage Casserole

(Ready in about 8 hours | Servings 12)

Ingredients

- 1 ½ cups spicy sausage

- 1 red onion, chopped

- 2 garlic cloves, smashed

- 1 sweet bell pepper, thinly sliced

- 1 jalapeño pepper

- 1/4 cup fresh parsley

- 1 heaping tablespoon fresh cilantro

- 1 (30-ounce) package hash brown potatoes, shredded and thawed

- 1 1/2 cups sharp cheese, shredded

- 1 cup milk

- 12 eggs

- 1 teaspoon dry mustard

- 1 teaspoon celery seeds

- 1/2 teaspoon salt

- 1/8 teaspoon pepper

- 1/4 teaspoon cayenne pepper

Directions

1. In a non-stick medium skillet, over medium flame, cook sausage; drain and set aside.

2. In a medium-sized bowl, combine onions, garlic, sweet bell pepper, jalapeño pepper, parsley and cilantro. Stir well to combine.

3. Alternate layers. Lay 1/3 of the hash browns, sausage, onion mixture and cheese into the crock pot. In the same way, repeat layers twice.

4. In a separate bowl, beat the rest of ingredients. Pour this mixture into the crock pot by spreading equally.

5. Cover and cook on low approximately 8 hours or overnight. Serve warm.

Sunrise Pork Sandwiches

(Ready in about 8 hours | Servings 12)

Ingredients

- 1 medium-sized pork butt roast

- 1/4 teaspoon black pepper

- 1/4 teaspoon crushed red pepper flakes

- 1 teaspoon sea salt

- 1 teaspoon dried thyme

- 1 tablespoon liquid smoke flavouring

- 12 pretzel buns

Directions

1. Pierce pork with a carving fork for better slow-cooking.

2. Season with spices and then spread liquid smoke over pork butt roast.

3. Lay pork roast into a crock pot.

4. Cover and cook on Low for 8 to 10 hours, turning once or twice.

5. Shred cooked pork roast, adding drippings to moisten. Make sandwiches with pretzel buns and enjoy!

Beer Pulled Pork Sandwiches

(Ready in about 10 hours | Servings 16)

Ingredients

- 1 medium-sized pork butt roast

- 1 large-sized onion, chopped

- 3 cloves garlic, smashed

- 2 carrots, thinly sliced

- 1/2 teaspoon ground black pepper

- 1/2 teaspoon cayenne pepper

- 1 teaspoon sea salt

- 1 teaspoon ground black pepper

- 1 teaspoon cumin powder

- 1 (12 fluid ounce) can beer

- 1 cup barbeque sauce

Directions

1. Pierce pork with a carving fork.

2. Put all of the ingredients, except barbeque sauce, into a crock pot.

3. Set crock pot to high; cook for 1 hour. Then reduce the heat to low and cook 6 to 8 hours longer.

4. Shred the cooked pork and return it to the crock pot. Add barbeque sauce and cook an additional 1 hour.

5. Serve on your favourite hamburger buns and enjoy!

Mom's Apple Crisp

(Ready in about 3 hours | Servings 6)

Ingredients

- 2/3 cup old-fashioned oats

- 2/3 cup brown sugar, packed

- 2/3 cup all-purpose flour

- 1 teaspoon allspice

- 1 teaspoon cinnamon

- 1/2 cup butter

- 5-6 tart apples, cored and sliced

Directions

1. In a medium-sized mixing bowl, combine together first six ingredients. Mix until everything is well blended.

2. Place sliced apples in your crock pot.

3. Sprinkle oat mixture over apples in the crock pot.

4. Cover the crock pot with three paper towels. Set the crock pot to high and cook for about 3 hours.

Vegetarian Quinoa with Spinach

(Ready in about 3 hours | Servings 4)

Ingredients

- 2 tablespoons olive oil

- 3/4 cup spring onions, chopped

- 1 cup spinach

- 2 garlic cloves, minced

- 1 cup quinoa, rinsed

- 2 ½ cups vegetable broth

- 1 cup water

- 1 tablespoon fresh basil

- 1 tablespoon fresh cilantro

- 1/4 teaspoon ground black pepper

- Salt to taste

- 1/3 cup Parmesan cheese

Directions

1. In a saucepan, heat olive oil over medium-high flame. Sauté spring onions, spinach and garlic until tender and fragrant. Transfer to a crock pot.

2. Add remaining ingredients, except the cheese, and cover with a lid.

3. Cook on LOW for about 3 hours.

4. Stir in Parmesan cheese, taste and adjust the seasonings; serve!

Easy Cheesy Quinoa with Veggies

(Ready in about 3 hours | Servings 4)

Ingredients

- 2 tablespoons margarine, melted

- 1 medium-sized onion, chopped

- 1 garlic clove, minced

- 1 cup button mushrooms, sliced

- 1 sweet red bell pepper

- 1 cup quinoa, rinsed

- 2 cups vegetable broth

- 1 ½ cup water

- 1 heaping tablespoon fresh parsley

- 1 heaping tablespoon fresh cilantro

- 1/4 teaspoon crushed red pepper flakes

- A pinch of ground black pepper

- Salt to taste

• 1/3 cup Parmesan cheese

Directions

1. In a medium-sized skillet, heat margarine over medium heat.

2. Sauté onions, garlic, mushrooms and red bell pepper in hot margarine for about 6 minutes or until just tender. Replace to a crock pot.

3. Add the rest of ingredients, except Parmesan cheese; set the crock pot to low and cook for about 3 hours.

4. Add Parmesan cheese and enjoy warm!

Kale Frittata with Sausages

(Ready in about 3 hours | Servings 6)

Ingredients

- Non-stick cooking spray

- 3/4 cup kale

- 1 sweet red bell pepper, sliced

- 1 sweet green pepper, sliced

- 1 medium-sized red onion, sliced

- 8 eggs, beaten

- 1/2 teaspoon ground black pepper

- 1 teaspoon salt

- 1 1/3 cup sausages

Directions

1. Combine all ingredients in a well-greased crock pot.

2. Set the crock pot to low and cook until frittata is set or about 3 hours.

3. You can reheat this frittata in microwave for 60 seconds.

Delicious Weekend Frittata

(Ready in about 3 hours | Servings 6)

Ingredients

- Non-stick cooking spray

- 1 1/3 cup cooked ham

- 1 red bell pepper, sliced

- 1 sweet green bell pepper, sliced

- 1 spring onions, sliced

- 8 eggs, beaten

- 1 tablespoon basil

- 1 heaping tablespoon fresh cilantro

- 1 tablespoon fresh parsley

- 1 teaspoon salt

- 1/4 teaspoon ground black pepper

- 1/4 teaspoon cayenne pepper

- A few drops of tabasco sauce

Directions

1. Grease a crock pot with non-stick cooking spray. Combine all ingredients in the crock pot.

2. Set the crock pot to low and cook your frittata approximately 3 hours.

3. Divide among six serving plates and sprinkle with chopped chives, if desired; garnish with sour cream and serve!

Vegetarian Breakfast Delight

(Ready in about 4 hours | Servings 4)

Ingredients

- 2 tablespoons canola oil

- 1 cup scallions, chopped

- 1 garlic clove, minced

- 2 medium-sized carrots, thinly sliced

- 1 celery stalk, chopped

- 1 cup quinoa, rinsed

- 2 cups vegetable stock

- 1 ½ cup water

- 1 tablespoon fresh cilantro

- A pinch of ground black pepper

- 1/4 teaspoon dried thyme

- 1/4 teaspoon dried dill weed

- Salt to taste

- 1/3 cup Parmesan cheese

Directions

1. In a medium-sized skillet, heat canola oil over medium heat.

2. Sauté scallions, garlic, carrots and celery for about 5 minutes, or until the vegetables are just tender. Transfer the vegetables to a crock pot.

3. Add quinoa, vegetable stock, water, cilantro, black pepper, dried thyme, dill weed and salt to taste.

4. Cover and cook on LOW approximately 4 hours.

5. Scatter Parmesan on top and serve warm!

Protein Rich Bacon Frittata

(Ready in about 4 hours | Servings 6)

Ingredients

- Non-stick cooking spray

- 1 cup scallions, sliced

- 1 1/3 cup bacon

- 1 cup mushrooms, sliced

- 1 poblano pepper, minced

- 10 eggs, beaten

- 1 heaping tablespoon fresh cilantro

- 1 teaspoon salt

- 1/4 teaspoon ground black pepper

- 1/4 teaspoon crushed red pepper flakes

Directions

1. Combine all of the ingredients in greased crock pot.

2. Next, set your crock pot to low; cover and cook the frittata 3 to 4 hours.

3. Cut into six wedges, garnish with mustard and serve!

Chili Mushroom Omelette

(Ready in about 4 hours | Servings 4)

Ingredients

- Non-stick cooking spray

- 1 green onions, sliced

- 2 cloves garlic, minced

- 2 cups mushrooms, sliced

- 1 chilli pepper, minced

- 2 ripe tomatoes, sliced

- 8 eggs, beaten

- 1 tablespoon fresh cilantro

- 1 teaspoon salt

- 1/4 teaspoon ground black pepper

- 1/4 teaspoon cayenne pepper

Directions

1. In your crock pot, place all of the ingredients.

2. Cover with a lid; cook on low 3 to 4 hours.

3. Cut into wedges and serve warm with sour cream and catsup.

Banana Pecan Oatmeal

(Ready in about 8 hours | Servings 4)

Ingredients

- 2 cups water

- 2 ripe bananas

- 1 cup steel-cut oats

- 1/4 cup pecans, coarsely chopped

- 2 cups soy milk

- 1/2 teaspoon cinnamon

- 1 teaspoon pure almond extract

- A pinch of salt

- Honey to taste

Directions

1. Pour water into your crock pot. Use an oven safe bowl (glass casserole dish works here) and place it inside your crock pot.

2. Mash the bananas with a fork or blend them in a blender. Transfer to the oven safe bowl.

3. Add remaining ingredients to the bowl.

4. Cook on low overnight or for 8 hours.

5. Stir well before serving and add toppings of choice. Enjoy!

Hearty Oatmeal with Nuts

(Ready in about 8 hours | Servings 4)

Ingredients

- 1 large-sized ripe banana

- 1 cup steel-cut oats

- 1/4 cup walnuts, coarsely chopped

- 2 tablespoons chia seeds

- 1 tablespoon hemp seeds

- 2 cups milk

- 1/4 teaspoon grated nutmeg

- 1/2 teaspoon cardamom

- 1/2 teaspoon cinnamon

- 1 teaspoon pure vanilla extract

- 2 cups water

- Maple syrup for garnish

- Fresh fruits for garnish

Directions

1. Mash banana with a fork. Add mashed banana to an oven proof dish. Stir in remaining ingredients.

2. Pour water into a crock pot.

3. Place the oven proof dish inside the crock pot. Cook on low heat setting overnight or for 8 hours. Top with maple syrup and fresh fruit.

Tomato Artichoke Frittata

(Ready in about 2 hours | Servings 4)

Ingredients

- Non-stick cooking spray

- 6 large-sized eggs, beaten

- 1 cup chopped artichoke hearts

- 1 medium-sized tomato, chopped

- 1 red bell pepper, chopped

- 1 teaspoon onion powder

- 1 teaspoon garlic powder

- 1/4 teaspoon ground black pepper

- 1/4 teaspoon cayenne pepper

- 1/4 cup Swiss cheese, grated

Directions

1. Coat a crock pot with cooking spray.

2. Add all of the ingredients to the crock pot.

3. Cover with a lid and cook on low-heat setting for about 2 hours.

4. Sprinkle with cheese; let stand for a few minutes until the cheese is melted.

Sausage Mushroom Omelette Casserole

(Ready in about 3 hours | Servings 4)

Ingredients

- 1 pound chicken breast sausage, sliced

- 1 cup scallions, chopped

- 1 cup mushrooms, sliced

- 4 medium-sized eggs

- 1 cup whole milk

- 1 teaspoon sea salt

- 1/4 teaspoon ground black pepper

- 1/2 teaspoon dry mustard

- 1/2 teaspoon granulated garlic

- 1/2 cup Swiss cheese, grated

Directions

1. Arrange sausage in a crock pot. Then, place scallions and mushrooms over the sausages.

2. In a mixing bowl, whisk together eggs, milk, and spices. Whisk to combine.

3. Cook on low-heat setting about 3 hours. Then spread cheese on top and allow to melt.

4. Serve warm with mayonnaise and mustard.

Pumpkin Pie Steel Cut Oats

(Ready in about 8 hours | Servings 4)

Ingredients

- 1 cup steel-cut oats

- 3 cups water

- 1/4 teaspoon ground cinnamon

- 1 cup pumpkin purée

- 1 teaspoon vanilla extract

- A pinch of salt

- 1 tablespoon pumpkin pie spice

- 1/2 cup maple syrup

Directions

1. Combine all ingredients in your crock pot.

2. Cover and cook on low overnight or for 8 hours.

3. Serve warm with raisins or dates, if desired!

Cocoa Steel Cut Oats

(Ready in about 8 hours | Servings 4)

Ingredients

- 3 ½ cups water

- 1 cup steel-cut oats

- 1/4 teaspoon grated nutmeg

- 1/2 teaspoon ground cinnamon

- 3 tablespoons cocoa powder, unsweetened

- A pinch of salt

- 1/2 teaspoon pure vanilla extract

- 1/2 teaspoon pure hazelnut extract

Directions

1. Add all of the ingredients to your crock pot.

2. Cook on low heat settings overnight or for 8 hours.

3. Stir before serving and add natural sweetener, if desired.

Nutty Pumpkin Oatmeal with Cranberries

(Ready in about 9 hours | Servings 4)

Ingredients

- 1 cup steel-cut oats

- 3 cups water

- 1 cup whole milk

- A pinch of salt

- 1 tablespoon pumpkin pie spice

- 1/2 teaspoon cardamom

- 1/4 cup pumpkin purée

- 2 tablespoons honey

- 1/2 cup dried cranberries

- 1/2 cup almonds, coarsely chopped

Directions

1. In a crock pot, place steel-cut oats, water, milk, salt, pumpkin pie spice, cardamom pumpkin purée, and honey.

2. Cook overnight or 8 to 9 hours.

3. Divide among serving bowls; sprinkle with dried cranberries and almonds; serve.

Cocoa Oatmeal with Bananas

(Ready in about 8 hours | Servings 4)

Ingredients

- 3 cups water

- 1 cup milk

- 1 cup steel-cut oats

- 1/2 teaspoon ground cinnamon

- 1 banana, mashed

- 4 tablespoons cocoa powder, unsweetened

- 1/2 teaspoon pure vanilla extract

- 1 banana, sliced

- Chopped pecans for garnish

Directions

1. Pour water and milk into a crock pot. Then place steel-cut oats, cinnamon, mashed banana, cocoa powder, and vanilla.

2. Set your crock pot to low and cook overnight or for 8 hours.

3. Stir before serving time; divide among serving bowls; garnish with banana and pecans and enjoy.

Cheese and Ham Quiche

(Ready in about 2 hours | Servings 4)

Ingredients

- Butter flavour non-stick cooking spray

- 4 slices of whole-wheat bread, toasted

- 2 cups sharp cheese, grated

- 1/2 pound ham, cooked and cut into bite-sized cubes

- 6 large-sized eggs

- 1/2 teaspoon Dijon mustard

- 1 cup heavy cream

- 1/4 teaspoon turmeric powder

- 1 tablespoon fresh parsley, coarsely chopped

- 1/2 teaspoon sea salt

- 1/4 teaspoon crushed red pepper

- 1/4 teaspoon freshly ground black pepper

Directions

1. Generously grease the inside of a crock pot with non-stick cooking spray.

2. Grease each slice of toasted bread with non-stick cooking spray; tear greased bread into pieces; arrange in the crock pot.

3. Spread 1/2 of the sharp cheese over the toast, and then place the cooked ham pieces over the cheese; top with the remaining cheese.

4. In a medium-sized mixing bowl or a measuring cup, beat the eggs together with the rest of ingredients; pour this mixture into the crock pot.

5. Cover and cook on high-heat setting for 2 hours. Serve warm with mayonnaise or sour cream, if desired.

Country Sausage and Cauliflower Breakfast

(Ready in about 6 hours | Servings 8)

Ingredients

- 1 pound sausage

- Non-stick spray

- 1 cup condensed cream of potato soup

- 1 cup whole milk

- 1 teaspoon dry mustard

- Salt to taste

- 1/2 teaspoon freshly ground black pepper

- 1 tablespoon fresh basil or 1 teaspoon dried basil

- 1 (28-ounce) package frozen hash browns, thawed

- 1 cup cauliflower, broken into florets

- 1 cup carrots, sliced

- 1/2 cup Cheddar cheese, shredded

Directions

1. In a cast-iron skillet, brown the sausage; cut into bite-sized chunks.

2. Coat the inside of the crock pot with non-stick spray. Add all ingredients, except Cheddar cheese; gently stir to combine.

3. Cover with a lid and cook for about 6 hours on low. Scatter Cheddar cheese on top. Let sit for 30 minutes before serving.

Broccoli Sausage Casserole

(Ready in about 6 hours | Servings 6)

Ingredients

- 2 tablespoons olive oil

- 3/4 pound sausage

- 1 cup beef broth

- 1 cup milk

- 1 teaspoon dry mustard

- 1/4 teaspoon cayenne pepper

- 1/2 teaspoon black pepper

- 2 pounds frozen hash browns, thawed

- 1 cup broccoli, broken into florets

- 1 cup carrots, sliced

- 1/2 cup Cheddar cheese, shredded

Directions

1. Coat the inside of the crock pot with olive oil.

2. In a medium-sized saucepan, over medium-high heat, cook the sausages until they are no longer pink or about 10 minutes. Transfer the sausage to the greased crock pot.

3. Add in broth, milk, mustard, cayenne pepper, black pepper, hash browns, broccoli and carrot. Cook on low for 6 hours.

4. Next, top with shredded cheese and allow to melt.

5. Serve warm with your favourite mayonnaise and some extra mustard.

Winter Morning Sausage and Vegetables

(Ready in about 6 hours | Servings 6)

Ingredients

- Non-stick spray

- 3/4 pound highly-spiced sausage

- 1 large-sized onion

- 1 sweet green bell pepper

- 1 sweet red bell pepper, chopped

- 1 cup whole milk

- 1 cup vegetable or beef broth

- 1/2 teaspoon chili powder

- 1/2 teaspoon black pepper

- Sea salt to taste

- 2 pounds frozen hash browns, thawed

- 1/2 cup Cheddar cheese, shredded

Directions

1. Oil the inside of your crock pot with non-stick spray.

2. In a medium-sized skillet, cook the sausage about 10 minutes, until it's browned. Replace to the crock pot.

3. Stir in remaining ingredients, except Cheddar cheese.

4. Set the crock pot to low and cook about 6 hours.

5. Scatter Cheddar cheese on top. Serve warm!

Eggs Florentine with Oyster Mushroom

(Ready in about 2 hours | Servings 4)

Ingredients

- Non-stick spray

- 2 cups Monterey Jack cheese, shredded

- 1 cup Swiss chard

- 1 cup oyster mushroom, sliced

- 2-3 garlic cloves, smashed

- 1 small onion, peeled and diced

- 5 large-sized eggs

- 1 cup light cream

- Salt to taste

- 1/4 teaspoon ground black pepper

Directions

1. Treat the inside of the crock pot with non-stick spray. Spread 1 cup of the Monterey Jack cheese over the bottom of the crock pot.

2. Then lay the spinach on top of the cheese.

3. Next, add the oyster mushroom in a layer. Top the mushroom layer with the garlic and onion.

4. In a measuring cup or a mixing bowl, beat the eggs with remaining ingredients. Pour this mixture over the layers in the crock pot.

5. Top with the remaining 1 cup of cheese.

6. Set your crock pot to high, cover with a lid and cook for 2 hours.

Cheese and Swiss chard Casserole

(Ready in about 4 hours | Servings 4)

Ingredients

- Butter flavour non-stick cooking spray

- 4 large-sized eggs

- 1 cup cottage cheese

- 3 tablespoons all-purpose flour

- 1 tablespoon fresh cilantro

- 1/2 teaspoon sea salt

- 1/4 teaspoon freshly ground black pepper

- 1/2 teaspoon dried thyme

- 1/2 teaspoon baking soda

- 2 tablespoons butter, melted

- 1 cup sharp cheese, grated

- 1 cup scallions, finely chopped

- 1 cup Swiss chard

Directions

1. Coat a heatproof casserole dish with cooking spray. Pour 2 cups of water into the crock pot.

2. Add the eggs and whisk them until frothy. Next, stir in the cottage cheese.

3. Add the flour, cilantro, sea salt, black pepper, thyme, baking soda, and butter. Mix well until everything is well incorporated.

4. Next, stir in remaining ingredients; adjust the seasonings.

5. Place the heatproof casserole dish onto the cooking rack in the crock pot; cover with a suitable lid and cook on low-heat setting approximately 4 hours.

6. Let cool to room temperature before serving time and enjoy!

Nutty Banana Frittata

(Ready in about 18 hours | Servings 6)

Ingredients

- 1 tablespoon canola oil

- 1 loaf bread, cut into cubes

- 1 cup cream cheese

- 2 ripe bananas

- 1 cup almonds, coarsely chopped

- 10 large eggs

- 1/4 cup maple syrup

- 1 cup half-and-half

- A pinch of salt

Directions

1. Grease the inside of your crock pot with canola oil.

2. Place 1/2 of bread cubes in the bottom of the crock pot. Then, evenly spread 1/2 of the cream cheese.

3. Arrange the slices of 1 banana over the cream cheese. Then scatter 1/2 of the chopped almonds.

4. Repeat the layers one more time.

5. In a mixing bowl or a measuring cup, whisk the eggs together with maple syrup, half-and-half and salt; pour over the layers in the crock pot.

6. Set in a refrigerator at least 12 hours. After that, cover and cook on low for 6 hours. Serve with some extra bananas if desired.

Yummy Spiced Pumpkin Frittata

(Ready in about 6 hours | Servings 6)

Ingredients

- 2 tablespoons coconut oil, melted

- 1 loaf bread, cut into small cubes

- 1 cup cream cheese

- 1 cup pumpkin, shredded

- 2 bananas, sliced

- 1 cup walnuts, coarsely chopped

- 8 eggs

- 1 cup half-and-half

- 2 tablespoons raw honey

- 1/2 teaspoon ground cinnamon

- 1/4 teaspoon grated cardamom

- 1/2 teaspoon allspice

- 1 teaspoon of pumpkin spice

• Powdered sugar for garnish

Directions

1. Coat the inside of a crock pot with coconut oil.

2. Place 1/2 of bread in the crock pot. Then, place 1/2 of the cream cheese.

3. Next, evenly spread 1/2 of shredded pumpkin. Lay the slices of 1 banana over the pumpkin. Scatter 1/2 of the chopped walnuts over the bananas.

4. Repeat the layers one more time.

5. In a medium-sized mixing bowl, whisk the eggs with the rest of ingredients, except powdered sugar. Pour this mixture over the layers in your crock pot.

6. Cook covered for 6 hours on low-heat setting. Dust your frittata with powdered sugar and serve!

Spiced Porridge for Busy Mornings

(Ready in about 8 hours | Servings 8)

Ingredients

- 2 cups steel-cut oats

- 6 cups water

- 2 cups milk

- 1 tablespoon pure orange juice

- 1 cup dried apricots, chopped

- 1 cup dates, chopped

- 1 cup raisins, chopped

- 1/2 teaspoon ginger

- 1 teaspoon ground cinnamon

- 1/8 teaspoon cloves

- 1/4 cup maple syrup

- 1/2 vanilla bean

Directions

1. Combine all of the ingredients in a crock pot.

2. Set the crock pot to low and leave overnight.

3. In the morning, stir prepared porridge, scraping the sides and bottom. Serve with jam or leftover eggnog, if desired.

Family Mid-Winter Porridge

(Ready in about 9 hours | Servings 8)

Ingredients

- 7 cups water

- 2 cups steel-cut Irish oats

- 1 teaspoon lemon zest

- 1 cup raisins

- 1 cup dried cranberries

- 1 cup dried cherries

- 1 tablespoon shredded coconut

- 1/2 teaspoon ginger

- 1 teaspoon allspice

- 1/8 teaspoon grated nutmeg

- 1/4 cup honey

- 1/2 vanilla bean

Directions

1. Place all ingredients in a crock pot; set crock pot to low.

2. Cook overnight or 8 to 9 hours.

3. Tomorrow, stir the porridge and divide among eight serving bowls. Serve with a dollop of whipped cream and roasted nuts, if desired.

Amazing Apple Oatmeal with Prunes

(Ready in about 7 hours | Servings 8)

Ingredients

- 2 cups steel-cut oats

- 1 cup apple juice

- 5 cups water

- 1/2 cup dried apples

- 1/4 cup dried cranberries

- 1/4 cup prunes

- 1/4 cup maple syrup

- 1 teaspoon allspice

- A pinch of salt

Directions

1. Add all ingredients to a crock pot.

2. Set a crock pot to low; cook the oatmeal for about 7 hours.

3. Serve warm topped with heavy cream if desired.

Tropical Overnight Oatmeal

(Ready in about 8 hours | Servings 8)

Ingredients

- 2 cups steel-cut Irish oats

- 4 cups water

- 1 cup apple juice

- 1 tablespoon fresh orange juice

- 1⁄2 cup dried papaya

- 1/2 cup dried pineapple

- 1/4 cup dried mango

- 1/4 cup maple syrup

- 2 tablespoon coconut flakes

- A pinch of salt

Directions

1. Combine all of the ingredients in your crock pot.

2. Cover with a suitable lid; leave the oatmeal overnight or 7 to 8 hours.

3. Serve with milk or a dollop of whipped cream. Enjoy!

English Muffins with Tomato Topper

(Ready in about 2 hours | Servings 12)

Ingredients

- 2 tablespoons vegetable oil

- 2 large-sized red onions, chopped

- 1 (28-ounce) can crushed tomatoes

- 1 tablespoon Worcester sauce

- 1 teaspoon lemon zest

- 1 tablespoon fresh cilantro

- 1 tablespoon fresh basil, chopped

- 1 teaspoon sea salt

- 1/4 teaspoon ground black pepper

- 1 cup mozzarella cheese

- 12 English muffins

Directions

1. In a medium-sized heavy skillet, heat vegetable oil over medium-high heat. Reduce the heat and then add onions. Sauté red onions until they are tender and translucent.

2. Transfer to the crock pot. Add in tomatoes and Worcester sauce. Cook covered on high for 1 hour or until the mixture begins to bubble around the edges.

3. Add remaining ingredients, except English muffins, and cook 1 hour longer. Serve warm with toasted English muffins.

Southern Creamy Grits

(Ready in about 8 hours | Servings 12)

Ingredients

- 1 ½ cups stone-ground grits

- 1 tablespoon butter

- 1/4 teaspoon turmeric powder

- 4 cups vegetable broth

- 1⁄2 teaspoon ground black pepper

- 1/2 teaspoon fine sea salt

- 1/2 cup sharp cheese, shredded

Directions

1. Combine all of the ingredients, except cheese, in your crock pot.

2. Cook on low-heat setting for 8 hours or overnight.

3. Add cheese to the prepared grits and enjoy. You can serve with eggs and bacon, if desired.

Grandma's Grits with Parmesan cheese

(Ready in about 9 hours | Servings 8)

Ingredients

- 2 cups stone-ground grits

- 1 tablespoon butter

- 1 teaspoons salt

- 1/2 teaspoon black pepper

- 1/2 teaspoon white pepper

- 1/4 cup heavy cream

- 1/2 cup freshly grated Parmesan cheese

Directions

1. Add all ingredients, except heavy cream and Parmesan cheese, to your crock pot.

2. Cook on low 8 to 9 hours.

3. In the morning, stir in heavy cream and Parmesan cheese; serve with your favourite topping and enjoy!

Super Greens and Bacon Casserole

(Ready in about 2 hours | Servings 6)

Ingredients

- 1 cup low-fat sharp cheese, shredded

- 1 cup leafy greens (such as spinach, kale, Swiss chard)

- 1/2 cup bacon, sliced

- 3 slices of bread, cubed

- 1 cup mushrooms, sliced

- 6 eggs

- 1/4 teaspoon black pepper

- 1/4 teaspoon cayenne pepper

- 1/2 teaspoon kosher salt

- 1 cup evaporated milk

- 1 cup vegetable broth

- 1 medium-sized onion

Directions

1. Spread half of the cheese on the bottom of the crock pot. Top with a layer of leafy greens. Next, lay 1/2 of the bacon.

2. Add the bread cubes and then place the mushrooms.

3. Add the remaining bacon and top with the remaining cheese.

4. In a measuring cup or a mixing bowl, combine the rest of ingredients. Pour this mixture into the crock pot.

5. Cook for 2 hours on high-heat setting. Divide among six serving plates and enjoy!

Delicious Wheat Berries

(Ready in about 10 hours | Servings 6)

Ingredients

- 1 ½ cups wheat berries

- 4 cups water

- 1/2 cup dried cranberries

- 1/2 vanilla bean

- Brown sugar for garnish

Directions

1. In a crock pot, place wheat berries, water, dried cranberries, and vanilla bean.

2. Stir to combine and cook for 8 to 10 hours.

3. Stir before serving, sprinkle with sugar and enjoy!

Multigrain Cereal Breakfast

(Ready in about 8 hours | Servings 6)

Ingredients

- 1/2 cup long-grain rice

- 1/2 cup wheat berries

- 1 cup rolled oats

- 1/2 teaspoon kosher salt

- 4 cups water

- Butter for garnish

Directions

1. Put rice, wheat berries, rolled oats, salt and water into a crock pot.

2. Cook, covered approximately 8 hours.

3. Stir before serving, add butter and enjoy!

Cereal with Fruit and Peanut Butter

(Ready in about 8 hours | Servings 6)

Ingredients

- 1/2 cup wheat berries

- 1 cup Irish-style oats

- 1/2 cup basmati rice

- 1/4 cup brown sugar

- 1/4 teaspoon ground cinnamon

- 4 cups water

- 1 cup dried fruit of choice

- Peanut butter for garnish

Directions

1. Place wheat berries, oats, basmati rice, sugar, cinnamon and water in your crock pot; stir to combine.

2. Cook for about 8 hours.

3. Divide among six serving bowls; garnish with dried fruit and peanut butter and serve.

Cheesy Spinach Quiche

(Ready in about 3 hours | Servings 6)

Ingredients

- Non-stick cooking spray

- 4 eggs

- 1/2 cup sharp cheese, shredded

- 3/4 cup baby spinach

- 2-3 cloves garlic, minced

- 1/4 cup green onion, chopped

- 1/2 teaspoon sea salt

- 1/2 teaspoon black pepper

- 1/2 teaspoon cayenne pepper

- 1 ½ cups evaporated milk

- 2 slices whole grain bread, cubed

Directions

1. Lightly grease your crock pot with cooking spray.

2. In a medium-sized mixing bowl, combine the eggs, cheese, spinach, garlic, onion, salt, black pepper, cayenne pepper and evaporated milk. Stir until everything is well incorporated.

3. Arrange the bread cubes on the bottom of the crock pot. Pour the egg-cheese mixture over the bread cubes.

4. Cover with a lid; cook for about 3 hours on high. Serve warm.

Cream of Broccoli and Cauliflower Soup

(Ready in about 4 hours | Servings 6)

Ingredients

- 1 cup water

- 2 cups reduced-sodium chicken broth

- 1 pound cauliflower, broken into florets

- 1 pound broccoli, broken into florets

- 1 yellow onion, finely chopped

- 3 cloves garlic, minced

- 1 heaping tablespoon fresh basil

- 1 heaping tablespoon fresh parsley

- 1/2 cup 2% reduced-fat milk

- Salt to taste

- 1/4 teaspoon white pepper

- 1/4 teaspoon black pepper

- Croutons of choice

Directions

1. Place water, broth, cauliflower, broccoli, onion, garlic, basil and parsley in your crock pot.

2. Cook on high 3 to 4 hours.

3. Transfer the soup to the food processor; add milk and spices and blend until uniform and smooth. Taste and adjust the seasonings; serve with croutons.

Family Broccoli-Spinach Soup

(Ready in about 4 hours | Servings 6)

Ingredients

- 2 cups water

- 2 cups reduced-sodium vegetable broth

- 1 pound broccoli, broken into florets

- 1 cup green onions, chopped

- 3 cloves garlic, minced

- 1 heaping tablespoon fresh cilantro

- 1 heaping tablespoon fresh parsley

- 2 cups spinach

- Salt to taste

- 1/4 teaspoon black pepper

Directions

1. Combine together water, vegetable broth, broccoli, green onions, garlic, cilantro and parsley in a crock pot.

2. Cook on high 3 hours. Add spinach and spices and cook for 20 minutes longer.

3. Pour the soup into the food processor; process until smooth.

4. Serve chilled or at room temperature. Garnish with a dollop of sour cream and enjoy!

Delicious Cream of Asparagus Soup

(Ready in about 4 hours | Servings 6)

Ingredients

- 2 cups vegetable stock

- 1 cups water

- 2 pounds asparagus, reserving the tips for garnish

- 1 onion, finely chopped

- 1 teaspoon lemon zest

- 2 cloves garlic, minced

- 1 teaspoon dried marjoram

- 1 heaping tablespoon fresh parsley

- 1/2 cup whole milk

- 1/4 teaspoon white pepper

- Salt to taste

Directions

1. Place stock, water, asparagus, onion, lemon zest, garlic, marjoram and parsley in a crock pot.

2. Cook on high-heat setting for 3 to 4 hours.

3. Meanwhile, steam asparagus tips until crisp-tender.

4. Pour the soup into a food processor; add milk, salt and white pepper and blend until smooth.

5. Garnish with steamed asparagus tips and serve at room temperature. You can also set your soup in a refrigerator and garnish it chilled.

Creamy Cauliflower Potato Chowder

(Ready in about 4 hours | Servings 6)

Ingredients

- 3 cups stock

- 1 cup carrot, chopped

- 3 ½ cups potatoes, diced

- 3 cups cauliflower, chopped

- 4 small-sized leeks, white parts only, chopped

- 1 cup milk

- 2 tablespoons cornstarch

- 1 teaspoon dried basil

- Salt to taste

- Black pepper to taste

Directions

1. Combine first five ingredients in a crock pot; set the crock pot to high and 3 to 4 hours.

2. Stir in remaining ingredients and cook 2 to 3 minutes longer or until thickened.

3. Blend the soup in a food processor or a blender until desired consistency is reached.

4. Adjust the seasonings and serve with sour cream.